HOW A CAR ACCIDENT CAN DESTROY YOUR LIFE

Don't Wait!
Your Health Depends On It!

DR. BAO THAI, D.C.

DEDICATION

This book is dedicated to my patients that I have been able to help. Seeing their progression from injured to living life again has never gotten old.

It is my life's work to help heal!

Table of Contents

1

MY STORY

Growing up as a child, I always knew I wanted to help people. I never knew to what degree. Being the first-born child in the United States, my parents always had great dreams and aspirations for me. They wanted to me to a doctor.

One day life just hit me in the face. My mother suffered from severe chronic asthma. Her asthma got so bad, that it would hospitalize her. I remember going to my mom's doctors' appointments and wondering why on earth is she not getting better.

She went to all the best doctors and was always on medications, but never seemed to improve. Seeing my mom, with the inhaler everyday made me depressed. I just could not understand. Her doctors all seemed very nice and knowledgeable. They were always confident when they wrote her prescription. The problem was, she just never got well.

These memories are my driving force to help more patients. To make a real difference in their lives without medications that are not fixing the problem. I have devoted myself to always finding a better way for my patients.

Being in an auto accident is a very traumatic event in someone's life. It could have major ramifications, if it's not dealt with properly. I can't begin to tell you, of all the thousands of patients I have seen where their health problems started from a simple car accident.

I hope this book will help anyone who has been in an accident, to take the necessary steps so they can enjoy a normal pain free life.

2

AUTO ACCIDENTS AND CHIROPRACTIC

If you have been riding or driving in a car during your life, the odds are that you have been in an automobile accident. During a survey, it was found that over 25% of drivers were involved in an auto accident in a five-year period. In 2008, there were 10.2 million auto accidents in the United States injuring 2.4 million people. In fact, someone is injured by a car crash every 14 seconds, which is the leading cause of acquired disability nationwide. [1]

When the body is subjected to the forces that occur in a motor vehicle accident, there is always some level of injury sustained by the person involved. This type of injury is most commonly referred to as "whiplash". It is a common misconception that whiplash injury only involves the neck, when in fact the entire spine is often damaged. **The forces introduced into the spine during crashes at speeds as low as 3 to 5 miles per hour have been shown to cause significant damage to the supportive structures of the spine** (your neck muscles, ligaments, and discs).

What Is Whiplash

Whiplash is an extremely *rapid* extension and flexion of the neck that results in injuries to the vertebrae, nerves, discs, muscles, ligaments and tendons.

There are four phases of whiplash injury. During a rear-end car crash, your body goes through a rapid acceleration and deceleration. In fact, going through the four phases of whiplash take less than a second.

During the first phase, your car is pushed out from under you and your back is flattened against the seat. This force shoves your cervical spine upwards and compresses your discs and joints. Additionally, your head moves backwards, creating stress. Your headrest should help reduce the movement of your neck, but damage can still occur.

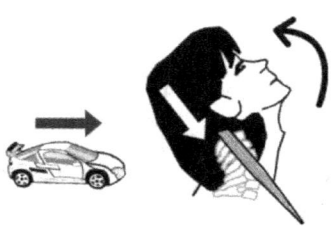

In phase two, your torso is accelerating faster than your vehicle but your head is still going backwards. This creates an S-curve in your cervical spine. During this same time, your seat is now recoiling forward acting like a springboard, causing your torso to move forward even more rapidly.

During the third phase, your torso comes to rest again in your seat, but your head and neck are accelerating forward creating an S-curve in the opposite direction.

During the fourth and final phase of whiplash, your torso is stopped by the seatbelt and your head continues to move forward with nothing to stop it. This results in a violent forward bending motion of your neck. This force can result in muscle strains and tears, in vertebrae being shoved out of their normal position, in the spinal cord being stretched and irritated, and even the brain hitting the inside of your skull.

Unlike broken bones or torn ligaments, an x-ray cannot detect whiplash, so it is much harder to diagnose and easier to go untreated. Newer imaging devices such as a CAT Scan, MRI, and ultrasound can show soft tissue injury, so it is essential if you've been in an accident that you seek treatment with someone who can provide these diagnostic tests.

The most common whiplash symptoms are:

- Neck pain and/or stiffness

- Blurred vision

- Difficulty swallowing

- Irritability

- Fatigue

- Dizziness

- Pain between the shoulder blades

- Pain in the arms or legs, feet and hands

- Headache

- Low back pain and/or stiffness

- Shoulder pain

- Nausea

- Ringing in the ears

- Vertigo

- Numbness and tingling

- Pain in the jaw or face

Injuries Resulting From Whiplash Trauma

Many factors determine the overall whiplash trauma that an individual will experience. It depends upon such things as:

- Direction of impact
- Speed of vehicles
- Sex
- Age
- Physical condition

Not only does whiplash look slightly different in each individual, but it also may take weeks or months to rear its ugly head. This is known as delayed onset whiplash.

Even though there is no prescribed pattern to whiplash, there are certain conditions that are common.

Neck Pain: Neck pain is the most common complaint when suffering from whiplash. Often this pain goes across the shoulders, up into the head and then down between the shoulder blades. Whiplash injuries tend to affect all of the tissues in the neck, including the facet joints, discs, as well as all of the muscles, ligaments and nerves.

Posterior Spinal Segment

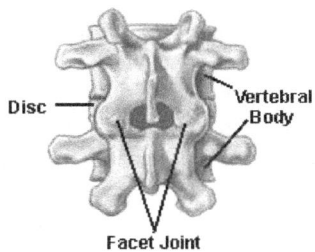

Disc — Vertebral Body

Facet Joint

The soreness you feel on the back of the neck, often to the right or left of center, is due to facet joint pain. This pain is typically tender to the touch. When you have pain due to the facet joint, your chiropractor will not be able to see it on an x-ray or MRI. Instead, your doctor will have to physically palpate the area to find the problem.

Disc injury tends to be the reason for chronic pain induced by whiplash. The outer wall of the disc (annulus) is made up of fibers that can easily be torn during a car accident. These tears lead to disc degeneration and herniations, which in turn, cause irritation and compression of the nerves running close to the disc. Once the degeneration or herniation has begun, your pain will move from being a neck pain to one that radiates into the arms, shoulders and upper back. You may even experience muscle weakness.

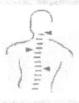 **Words Defined: Herniated Disc**

The gel-like inside of a spinal disc oozes out of the annulus and presses against a nerve causing severe pain.

The immediate pain that you feel after a car accident is often due to damaged muscles and ligaments. This damage causes stiffness and restricted motion. As the muscles heal, the pain lessens. However, the restricted movement may continue. Damage to the ligaments often results in abnormal movement and instability.

Headaches: Headaches are the next most common complaint from someone suffering a whiplash injury. Although some headaches are due to the brain hitting the skull during impact, many are due to injury to muscles, ligaments and facet joints of the cervical spine.

TMJ Dysfunction: TMJ is the temporomandibular joint or jaw joint along with the surrounding muscles. TMJ dysfunction can be quite painful, making it difficult to eat, swallow and yawn. Common symptoms of TMJ dysfunction include:

- Pain or tenderness

- Limited ability to open the mouth wide

- Jaws that get "stuck" in the open or closed position

- Clicking, popping or grating sounds

- Tired feeling in the face

- Difficulty chewing

- Sudden uncomfortable bite as if the upper and lower teeth are not fitting together properly

- Swelling on the side of the face

- Toothache

- Headache

- Neck ache

- Dizziness

- Earaches

- Hearing problems

If not properly evaluated and treated, TMJ problems can continue to worsen and lead to headaches, facial pain, ear pain and difficulty eating.

Brain Injury: The human brain is made up of soft tissue. This tissue is suspended in a watery substance known as cerebrospinal fluid. During an accident, as your head and neck are thrown first backward, then forward, then back again, your brain bounces off the skull and can lead to bruising and bleeding. Although it is possible to lose consciousness due to such an injury, most people remain conscious but report feeling confused or disoriented in the short term. In the long term, brain injury from whiplash can cause things such as:

- Mild confusion

- Difficulty concentrating
- Sleep disturbances
- Irritability
- Forgetfulness
- Loss of sex drive
- Depression
- Emotional instability

In fact, it is even possible that your sense of smell and taste, or even your vision is affected.

Dizziness: Dizziness is typically a result of injury to the facet joints of the spine, though it is possible that it results from a brain injury. Luckily, dizziness is a very temporary side effect of whiplash and can be easily treated with chiropractic.

Low Back Pain: Most people think of neck pain when they think of whiplash. Many of us have seen the neck collars worn by someone who was recently in a car accident. The lower back, however, is also prone to injury during the four phases of whiplash. In fact, low back pain is found in nearly one-half of all rear-end collisions and nearly 75 percent of all side impact crashes.[2] Why is the lower back subject to injury? Despite not having the large range of flexion and extension, the lower back still goes through tremendous compression. This compression causes injury to the discs, ligaments and muscles.

Substandard Treatment is Too Often the Norm for Whiplash Victims

In more cases than not, people involved in motor vehicle accidents receive substandard care for their injuries. Often when they are taken to the emergency room, not much is done unless the doctor suspects internal bleeding, head injury, fracture, or other life threatening conditions. The emergency room physicians simply are *not looking* for soft tissue injury like muscle or ligament tears. Even if x-rays of the spine *are* taken, the doctor is only looking for a fracture. He or she is NOT looking at the biomechanical integrity of the spine nor the muscles, ligaments, or discs for injury.

The doctor will usually prescribe anti-inflammatory drugs such as Motrin, Naproxin, and pain killers and leave the patient with the impression that if their soreness goes away within a few days to weeks, then they are better and no serious injury has occurred. *This could not be further from the truth!* Unfortunately, even if the pain goes away as predicted, the damage to the spine remains to make its presence known again another day, usually when the patient least expects it.

When the spine and the muscles and ligaments surrounding it are injured and left uncorrected, the problems worsen as time goes on. Most commonly, the patient's spine has a mechanical problem (Ex: abnormal positioning of the vertebra) that produces excessive wear and tear on the spinal joints. Over time, this abnormal position and the resultant stress it produces causes joint swelling, disc degeneration, scar tissue formation, and eventually arthritis.

In most cases, the cause of the person's pain is *directly* related to the abnormal positioning of their spine. Our techniques are the most modern approach to spinal rehabilitation available. The goal of our care is to restore normal (or to as near normal as possible) structure to your spine, and then also more normal function.

Chiropractic Care for Whiplash

It is essential to have a chiropractic evaluation of your spine and posture if you have *EVER* been involved in a car accident, no matter how long ago it was!

When you see your chiropractor after an auto accident, he will do a thorough evaluation of your entire spine. He will check your neck (cervical spine), your mid-back (thoracic spine) and your low back (lumbar spine). Although you may just have neck pain, any region of your spine may be affected.

What will your chiropractor be looking for?

- Restricted joint motion
- Disc injury
- Muscle spasm
- Ligament injury

**Studies Show
Chiropractic Is Best Therapy for Whiplash**

A study was undertaken to determine the effects of chiropractic in a group of 28 patients who had been referred with chronic 'whiplash' syndrome. The severity of patients' symptoms was assessed before and after treatment. Ninety-three percent of patients improved following chiropractic treatment [3]

Your chiropractor has a host of diagnostic tests that can help him determine where your problems lie. For instance, he will use motion and static palpations, which is an examination by means of touch. During the palpations, he will be checking for tenderness, tightness and movement.

Your chiropractor will also take a look at your overall posture and how you walk. This will help him determine whether your body mechanics are working properly.

Of course, your chiropractor will take x-rays to see if you have any degeneration or misalignment of the spine. These x-rays can also help your chiropractor determine if you need a CAT scan or an MRI for further diagnosis.

Once all the diagnostic tests have been done, your chiropractor will understand your unique case of whiplash and how best to help you with an effective treatment plan.

The Stages of Whiplash Treatment

In the initial intensive or relief care phase of chiropractic care for whiplash, the main goal is to get rid of your pain and stabilize your condition as quickly as possible.

Your chiropractor will concentrate on reducing inflammation by using ultrasound and/or gentle stretching and manual therapies. You may also use cold therapy or a neck support.

As your neck area becomes less inflamed, your chiropractor will begin to use spinal manipulation to help you return normal motion to your spinal joints.

The number of times you visit a chiropractor during the relief stage will vary based on your particular condition. Typically, however, this phase lasts from a week to a month, with visits three times per week.

Once you have passed through the relief stage, you will move on to the rehabilitative stage of therapy. During this phase, you will have begun participating in your normal activities again. However, if you do not continue treatment, your pain is likely to reappear because your condition has not yet been fully stabilized.

The goals of rehabilitative care include:

- Strength
- Flexibility
- Increased muscle control and coordination

- Increased balance
- Reducing fear and avoidance of normal activities

This phase of care can take a few weeks to several months, depending on the severity of your condition. Typically, the amount of care is not quite as frequent as relief care.

Treatment Approaches for Whiplash Injuries

The pain and restricted motion you experience after a whiplash injury is due to injured tissue. It is also due to the protective response of the nervous system. Your nervous system purposely locks up your spinal joints to protect you from injury to the spinal cord itself. It is your chiropractor's job to restore your injured tissues and unlock your spinal joints. Your treatment plan will depend entirely on your particular diagnosis. However, there are many traditional approaches used for whiplash. Let's discuss a few of them.

The most common treatment for whiplash is manual manipulation. Manual manipulation of the spine restores the normal movement and position of the vertebrae.

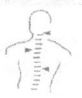 **Words Defined: Manual Manipulation**

Where the chiropractor moves a joint to the end of its range, and then applies a low-force thrust.

Manual manipulation is the most effective treatment for minimizing the long-term effects of whiplash. It is even more effective when used with massage therapy, trigger point therapy, exercise rehabilitation and other soft tissue rehabilitation therapies.[4]

Some spinal manipulation techniques are:

- Specific Spinal Manipulation: Your chiropractor will identify specific joints that show restricted motion, known as subluxations. He will return motion to the joint using a gentle thrusting motion. The gentle thrusting rapidly stretches the soft tissue as well as stimulates the nervous system.

- Flexion-Distraction Technique: This is a gentle manipulation that does not use any thrust. It is often used to treat bulging or herniated discs. Your chiropractor will use a special table to assist with this technique that uses a slow pumping action on the disc rather than a direct force.

- Instrument-Assisted Manipulation: This is another non-thrusting technique. To do this procedure, your chiropractor will use a hand-held instrument to apply force without thrusting the spine.

In addition to manipulation, your chiropractor may also use manual therapies. These therapies treat injured soft tissues such as ligaments and muscles.

Some examples of manual therapies include:

- Trigger Point Therapy: Your chiropractor will identify tight, painful points on a muscle. Once identified, your chiropractor will put direct pressure on these points with their fingers to relieve the tension.

- Manual Joint Stretching and Resistance Techniques: These are techniques that help to stretch out your joints against some form of resistance. One common resistant manual joint therapy technique is called muscle energy therapy. In this therapy, you will actively use your muscles in a specific direction while your chiropractor applies a counterforce to your movements.

- Therapeutic Massage: Therapeutic massage is the manual manipulation of the body's soft tissue, and is generally used for the reduction of stress and pain. This differs from "getting a massage" with the main goal of relaxation. Though you may feel relaxed after a therapeutic massage, the goal is the relief of pain.

- Instrument-Assisted Soft Tissue Therapy: Your chiropractor will perform repeated strokes with an instrument over the muscle injury area. These strokes are gentle and have a massage-like quality.

In addition to the different kinds of manual techniques available to your chiropractor, he may also treat your whiplash injury with other modalities. Some examples include:

- Interferential Current (IFC): The IFC machine produces electrical currents that pass through the affected area of the patient by placing two electrodes on the skin at a painful area or the spinal nerve root associated with a painful region. Alternating currents are applied and the currents rise and fall at different frequencies. These frequencies cause the body to produce endorphins, which stops the pain signals from reaching the brain.

- Ultrasound: Therapeutic ultrasound stimulates tissue below the skin's surface using sound waves. Essentially, it is a high frequency massage that goes below the surface of the skin.

- Therapeutic Exercises: These exercises improve the joint mechanics and return your spine to normal motion. Chiropractors commonly prescribe specific strengthening exercises for their patients with whiplash.

SOURCES:

1. US Census Bureau http://www.census.gov/compendia/statab/cats/transportation/motor_vehicle_accidents_and_fatalities.html.

2. McConnell WE, Howard RP, Guzman HM, et al. "Analysis of human test subject kinematic responses to low velocity rear end impacts." *SAE Tech Paper Series*. 1993.

3. Woodward MN, Cook JCH, Gargan MF, Bannister GC. "Chiropractic treatment of chronic whiplash injuries." *Injury*. 1996.

4. Cesar Fernandez de las Penas a, Luis Palomeque del Cerrob, Josue Fernandez Carneroa. "Manual treatment of post-whiplash injury."*Journal of Bodywork and Movement Therapies*. 2005.

3

WHEN ACCIDENTS HAPPEN...

What You Need To Know If You've Been In An Auto Accident

If you or a friend or loved one has been involved in an automobile accident, you need to know what to do about your health and welfare and you need to know what steps to take to document the accident. First, here's what you should know about your health.

1. Even a minor accident can cause injury. Never assume that you are not injured just because there is little or no damage to your car. Seek professional care immediately.
2. If a paramedic suggests you go to the emergency room, don't decline. You may be suffering from shock, and will be unable to properly judge the situation. Even the smallest fracture in your spine can be very serious!
3. Muscle aches, soreness, headaches and other symptoms associated with whiplash injuries may not show up until 24-72 hours after the accident. The sooner you seek treatment, the less likely it will be that you will have severe pain or permanent damage.
4. Studies show that ICE applied immediately to the injured area will help keep swelling and pain to a minimum.

We have covered a lot of the health issues and what happens to your body during an auto accident in our Auto Accidents and Chiropractic chapter. Please read it carefully so you understand how imperative it is that you do not ignore your body regardless of how you feel initially after any accident.

When you've had an accident or if a loved one has been involved in an accident you may be emotionally shaken and overwhelmed. Please read this chapter so you are prepared and informed as to what to do, should you ever need this advice.

When An Accident Has Occurred

Emergency Checklist

It's important to take care of certain items as soon as an accident occurs. Here is a checklist of what to do at the scene of the accident:

- Exchange insurance & contact information with the other driver(s)

- Document the driver's license number of other driver

- Document the license plate number of the other vehicle

- Call the local or state police department

- Get the names of all witnesses

- Document all damages to your vehicle (take photos with your cell phone if you can. Or keep a disposable camera in your glove compartment for an emergency like this)

- Draw a picture of the accident while it is fresh in your mind (see our diagram on the next page)

- List all important factors that may pertain to the accident (including if the other person was running a light, speeding, talking on a cell phone, etc.)

Accident Diagram:

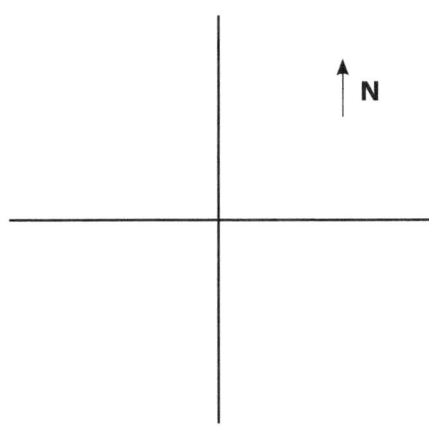

For your protection please be sure to include all the information you can. It is important to list all cars involved and their location and damage after the accident. You can use the map above to draw the details of your accident.

Witness Name   Phone Number

_____

_____

_____

_____

Other important facts about the accident:

_____

_____

_____

_____

_____

_____

_____

In order to be prepared you should have these phone numbers and corresponding information saved in your cell phone, or you should keep a list written out in your glove compartment so that they are easy to access,. This will make it easier for you to access if you are in an emotional state of stress:

__Important Numbers and Information__

Chiropractor	Dr. Bao Thai DC	940-312-6936
Insurance Agent		
Insurance Company		
Policy #		
Towing Company		
Nearest Relative		
Medical Doctor		
Car Rental		
Medical Information:		
Allergies:		
Medication Taken:		
Medical Conditions:		

4

THE THREE PHASES OF CHIROPRACTIC CARE

Like the building of a house, chiropractic does things in a certain order so that the spine can be strong and work correctly. For instance, when building a house, you must have a strong foundation before you try to put up walls. Equally as important, you must have walls before you add on the roof.

The same is true for your body. You must go through a plan of care in the right order so that it can heal itself fully and correctly.

There are three general phases of chiropractic care: the initial intensive or relief care; rehabilitation care; and wellness or maintenance care. Let's take a look at each.

Initial Intensive or Relief Care

For the most part, My patients come to our office because they have pain. In fact, more than 70% of our patients have specify back and neck problems as the health problem for which they are seeking chiropractic care.[1]

In the initial intensive or relief care phase of chiropractic care, the main goal is to get rid of your pain and stabilize your condition as quickly as possible. Since pain is usually the last symptom to show itself and the first to resolve itself, progress is seen very quickly.

The number of times you visit a chiropractor during the relief phase will vary based on your particular condition. Typically, however, this phase lasts from a week to a month, with visits three times per week.

Studies Show
Chiropractic Care Provides Relief to Patients

A majority of people who have used non-medical healthcare found a great deal of benefit from that care and were very satisfied. Chiropractic was one of the most common and successful alternative modalities used to treat back pain.[2]

Rehabilitative Care

The next phase is rehabilitative care. Do you believe that if you have no pain then you must be healthy? If so, you agree with most people, but like them, you would be wrong. Pain is a poor indicator of health and typically only appears after a disease or condition has been present a long time.

Let's look at a few examples. A cavity in your tooth only begins to hurt when it has hit the nerve. At that point, you are looking at some major dental work. When it was a simple cavity, you had no pain. Or perhaps you can think of diabetes. By the time a diabetic feels leg pain, the diabetes is causing poor circulation to the extremities, often leading to severe procedures such as amputation. An earlier diagnosis could have prevented this with medication.

What does this have to do with your spine? Pain in your spine usually means a problem has advanced. The reduction of pain is great, but does not mean the problem has been resolved. That is why you need rehabilitative care.

By the time you have reached the rehabilitative phase, you once again feel like participating in your normal activities. If you do so, however, without continued care, your pain is likely to reappear because your condition has not yet been fully stabilized.

The goals of rehabilitative care include:

- Strength
- Flexibility
- Increased muscle control and coordination
- Increased balance
- Reducing fear and avoidance of normal activities

This phase of care can take a few weeks to several months, depending on the severity of your condition. Typically, the amount of care is not quite as frequent as relief care.

However, it is important to realize that your condition may have taken years to develop, so it will take time to correct. For instance, the pain associated with low back pain may resolve easily with chiropractic. The problem is that recurrent episodes are common. This has been shown to be a problem in the multifidus muscle that cannot become strong and healed without rehabilitation.[3]

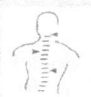 **Words Defined: Multifidus Muscle**

A thin muscle that spans three vertebrae of the spine that works to stabilize the joints.

> **Studies Show**
> **Rehabilitative Care Improves LBP**
>
> Thirty-nine patients with acute, first-episode LBP were either put into two random groups – one with rehabilitative care and one without. After one and three years of treatment, interviews were conducted. Rehabilitative therapy and the resumption of normal activity is more effective in reducing low back pain than just resuming normal activities alone.[4]

In addition to regular adjustments during the rehabilitative phase, care may be accompanied by rehabilitation exercises, nutrition and modification of daily habits.

Wellness Care

Once you have finished rehabilitative care, you then move on to the wellness phase. Your wellness program will be designed specifically for you and will include such things as good nutrition and exercise.

A good way to look at wellness care is to relate it to car care. We all know that it takes a long time for an engine to blow, but with regular maintenance, the car will run well for many years and many miles. Similarly, it takes a long time to develop subluxations in the spine. With regular wellness care, the vertebrae will not have a chance to get out of line. Treatment frequency can range from once per week to once every two months.

The goals of this phase of chiropractic care are:

- Improving health
- Encouraging normal spinal function
- Preventing the return of the original condition
- Catching small problems before they become serious

Wellness care is very important, especially given the state of health in the United States. Healthcare spending in the United States exceeded $2 trillion in 2006, and is projected to reach $4.2 trillion by 2017.[5] The problem is that most of this money doesn't go for "health" care but for "sick" care.

Studies Show
Chiropractic Care Results in Significant Savings

This study compared 75-year-old chiropractic patients with non-chiropractic patients. The study concluded that those receiving chiropractic care reported better overall health, spent fewer days in hospitals and nursing homes, used fewer prescription drugs and were more active than their counterparts. Additionally, chiropractic patients reported 21% less time in hospitals over a three-year period of time.[7]

Economist Paul Zane Pilzer summarized the situation well: "The sickness business is reactive. Despite its enormous size, people become customers only when they are stricken by and react to a specific condition or complaint ... the wellness business is proactive. People voluntarily become customers - to feel healthier, to reduce the effects of aging, and to avoid becoming customers of the sickness business. Everyone wants to be a customer of this earlier-stage approach to health."[6]

First Appointment

No matter why you start going to a chiropractor, whether it is for pain relief, stabilization of a problem or simply to stay well, you will go through an initial appointment. Here is what you can expect.

Paperwork: Your chiropractor will have you fill out paperwork designed to provide them with your health history and information on your current condition.

Consultation: Your first interaction with the chiropractor will be to discuss your concerns and issues. This helps your doctor learn more about you, your condition and your expectations. In this way, your doctor can determine how chiropractic can meet your goals.

Examination: After your consultation, the chiropractor will perform a complete physical examination including standard neurological, orthopedic, postural and chiropractic specific tests.

Further studies: Depending on your specific condition, you may get x-rays, or be referred for an MRI, CAT scan or other diagnostic test.

Report of findings: Once examination and testing is complete, you will receive a detailed report about the findings. You will also have the opportunity to ask any questions that you may have about the findings.

Discuss recommendations: At this point, your doctor will discuss a plan of action. He will show you what can be done for your condition and how he is going to accomplish your goals.

Treatment: This may include such things as adjustments.

Depending upon the treatment plan, you may get your first adjustment after the chiropractor go over your x-rays on your second visit

At Home: Prior to leaving, your chiropractor will suggest activities and plans of action for you to complete outside the office environment. This might include ice or heat application instructions, certain activities or positions to avoid and home exercises and/or stretches.

Whether you come into a chiropractor's office because you have pain or simply because you want to remain pain-free, you will get your own personalized plan of action. Following the plan will help you get healthy and stay that way.

SOURCES:

1. Coulter, ID, Hurwitz, EL, Adams, AH, Genovese BJ, Hays R, Shekelle, PG. "Patients using chiropractors in North America: who are they, and why are they in chiropractic care?" *Spine.* 1976.

2. **Kanodia, Anup K.** "Perceived Benefit of Complementary and Alternative Medicine for Back Pain" *The Journal of the American Board of Family Medicine.* 2010.

3. Hides, JA, Jull, GA, Richardson, CA. "Long-term effects of specific stabilizing exercises for first-episode low back pain." *Spine.* 2001.

4. Hides, JA, previously cited.

5. Keehan S, Sisko A, Truffler C, et al: "Health Spending Projections Through 2017: The Baby-Boom Generation is Coming to Medicare." *Health Affairs.* 2008.

6. Pilzer PZ. *The Wellness Revolution.* John Wiley and Sons. New York. 2002.

7. Coulter ID, Hurwitz EL, Aronow HU, et al. "Chiropractic patients in a comprehensive home-based geriatric assessment, follow-up and health promotion program." *Topics in Clinical Chiropractic.* 1996.

5

HELP, THE PAIN IS KILLING ME!

Proactive Approach to Pain

Many Americans suffer from chronic pain. In fact, according to the National Centers for Health Statistics, more than one-quarter of Americans (26%) age 20 years and over - an estimated 76.5 million Americans - report that they have had a problem with pain. They awaken in the morning in pain and go to bed at night in pain. And for many, sleep is interrupted due to pain. Such pain limits activities and limits life enjoyment. But what can a person do?

Stat Fact

An estimated 20% of American adults (42 million people) report that pain or physical discomfort disrupts their sleep a few nights a week or more. [1]

The old view solution was to see a medical doctor who would most likely prescribe pain medication. Of course, as time went on, more and more medication would be needed in order to combat the pain. And that was if you were lucky enough to be helped by the pain medication in the first place.

If the pain persisted, surgery was often the next avenue of care. The problem with surgery is that the "cure" often leaves chronic pain sufferers in more pain. Perhaps a different pain, but pain nonetheless.

The old medical model is a model of disease. The first line of defense is to mask the symptoms. The second line of defense is to surgically repair. This is very different from the wellness model practiced by chiropractors.

Chiropractors do not seek to mask symptoms. Instead, we seek to help the body function at its most optimal level by fixing subluxations in the spine. We seek the cause of the problem.

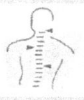 **Words Defined: Vertebral Subluxation**

An interference of the nervous system due to a misalignment and or abnormal motion of spinal vertebra which causes improper communication with associated organs, muscles and tissues of the body.

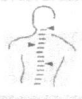 **Words Defined: Acute Pain**

Pain that comes on quickly, can be severe, but lasts a relatively short time.

In order to understand how chiropractic can help chronic pain sufferers, it will be helpful to define pain.

Pain is not a bad thing in and of itself. Of course for those experiencing it, it is no fun. However, pain is the body's way of sending an SOS to the body. The message is that something is wrong and the SOS is loud enough that it can't be ignored.

If a person feels a sufficient amount of pain, they will stop doing the activity that is causing the pain. This is the protective mechanism built into the body to help prevent further injury.

Pain is useful as long as it is keeping us healthy. However, pain can get out of control. It can continue long after its usefulness has been achieved.

Pain that stops you from injuring yourself further is called acute pain. It is the body's response to injury. For instance, if you twist your ankle while hiking along a trail, the pain you feel is acute pain. Chronic pain is that which persists far beyond the twisted ankle.

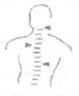 **Words Defined: Chronic Pain**

Pain that lasts long after the initial injury has healed. It may be caused by a disease, such as arthritis, or it may be the result of an injury such as back strain.

Chronic pain has many sources:

- Injuries that did not heal correctly or completely
- Long-term disease
- Injuries to the nervous system

Stat Fact

The annual cost of chronic pain in the United States, including healthcare expenses, lost income, and lost productivity, is estimated to be $100 billion. [2]

Of course, there are other potential sources, but no matter what, the source of chronic pain is one that encompasses an unresolved issue with the body.

The biggest problem with chronic pain is that it starts a vicious cycle that leads to more pain. The longer we feel pain, the more our body tries to accommodate the pain. This is often through unusual body movements and posture, and through a reduction of activities. The more the body accommodates the pain, the more difficult it is to get rid of it. It can be a very difficult cycle to break.

This is where chiropractic care comes in. Chiropractic treatment can help reduce or even eliminate many kinds of pain and has been shown to be especially effective with chronic pain.

Studies Show
Chiropractic More Effective Than
Medication or Acupuncture

The January 2005 issue of the Journal of Manipulative and Physiological Therapeutics showed that patients with chronic back pain did better with chiropractic than with medication or acupuncture, both during the 13-week treatment and 12 months later. At the 12-month mark, only those that received chiropractic care still had significant improvement. The conclusion: "Overall, patients who have chronic mechanical spinal pain syndromes and received spinal manipulation gained significant broad-based beneficial short-term and long-term outcomes." [3]

How can chiropractic help when medication cannot? Chiropractic principles state that although injury or illness may be the original cause of pain, everything that happens to the body involves the nervous system.

- Any impact to the body will involve the skeletal system in general and the spine in particular
- Disease causes muscular issues. Muscles affect the way we move. Movement and posture affects the spine.
- Blocked nerve impulses are due to subluxations in the spine.

Studies Show
Chiropractic Better Than Muscle
Relaxants for Low Back Pain

A study published in the July 2004 Journal of Manipulative and Physiological Therapeutics compared the effects of chiropractic adjustments to muscle relaxants in patients' low back pain that lasted two to 12 weeks. The three groups of patients included those with chiropractic adjustments and a placebo, those receiving muscle relaxants with fake adjustments, and finally a group with placebo medications and fake adjustments. The results showed for pain and severity, the chiropractic group did better than the other two groups. The conclusion: "Statistically, the chiropractic group responded significantly better than the control group with respect to a decrease in pain scores." [4]

Chiropractic's role is to establish the normal function of muscles, joints and the nervous system, thus eliminating the root causes of chronic pain.

Studies have shown that chiropractic treatments are among the most effective pain management plans. Chiropractic is low-risk. It has no side effects like those associated with medication. And best of all, chiropractic may not only manage pain, but can eliminate the cause of pain altogether.

Oh My Aching Back

Four out of five people initially come to a chiropractor because of back pain. Back pain can be caused by:

- Pinched nerves
- Bulging or herniated discs
- Scoliosis
- Arthritis
- Muscle pain
- Vertebral subluxation

The National Center for Complementary and Alternative Medicine in 2010 concluded that spinal manipulation/mobilization may be helpful for several conditions in addition to back pain, including:

- Migraine and cervicogenic (neck-related) headaches
- Neck pain
- Upper- and lower-extremity joint conditions
- And whiplash-associated disorders[5]

Stat Fact

Back pain is the leading cause of disability in Americans under 45 years old. More than 26 million Americans between the ages of 20-64 experience frequent back pain. [6]

For years, medical doctors have held the belief that lower back pain will resolve itself within three months with or without some kind of intervention. This is contrary, however, to what doctors of chiropractic have known to be true for years. In fact, a recent study in the British Medical Journal found that only one in four back pain sufferers had recovered 12 months after an initial visit to a medical doctor.

The Consumer Reports Health Rating Center released the results of a survey of over 14,000 patients with back pain on April 6, 2009. Results showed that chiropractic spinal manipulation is the top-rated treatment for people suffering with back pain. In fact, survey respondents were almost twice as likely to be highly satisfied with their chiropractic care than they were with their medical care.

**Studies Show
Chiropractic is Cost-Effective in
Treating Chronic Back Pain**

A study published in the October 2005 issue of The Journal of Manipulative and Physiological Therapeutics (JMPT) showed that chiropractic patients with both acute and chronic pain had less pain and higher satisfaction than those that sought medical care. Additionally, chiropractic treatment was 16 percent less expensive than medical care costs. And finally, the satisfaction rate among chiropractic patients was much higher. The conclusion: "With their mission to increase value and respond to patient preferences, health care organizations and policy makers need to reevaluate the appropriateness of chiropractic as a treatment option for low-back pain." [7]

Chiropractic spinal manipulation is effective for back pain and musculoskeletal injuries – based on both research and patient satisfaction. Using chiropractic for these problems should definitely be a first choice course of action, especially since we provide a drug-free, non-invasive, personalized treatment plan.

**Studies Show
Low Back Pain Study by Insurance
Company Favorable to Chiropractic**

Blue Cross/Blue Shield (BCBS) of Kansas presented a study titled "Lumbago Treatment." The results showed that chiropractic was more cost-effective than anesthesiology; neurosurgery; neurology; registered physical therapy; orthopedic reconstructive surgery; physical medicine and rehabilitation; and rheumatology. Patients had a willingness to return to the chiropractor that was 22% greater than the combined total of medical portals. The conclusion: "Patients suffering from back problems are better off with cost-effective chiropractic care." [8]

Don't Be a Pain In the Neck

Stat Fact

Neck pain is very common with approximately 15 percent of women and 10 percent of men affected at any given time. [9]

Your neck is also known as the cervical spine. It begins at the base of the skull and has seven tiny vertebrae. This small structure supports your head, which weighs 12 to 15 pounds. The miracle is that your cervical spine can move your head in every direction. That miracle of flexibility, however, makes you neck very susceptible to injury and pain. The study of how the neck and head move is called biomechanics.

One way that biomechanics affects the neck is through postural stress.

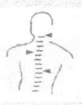 **Words Defined: Postural Stress**

Strain on the nerves, blood vessels and soft tissues from sitting for long hours or performing repetitive motions. This can lead to tight muscles, chronic soft tissue inflammation and arm symptoms.

In addition to long hours of sitting or performing repetitive motions, poor spinal mechanics, weak or overdeveloped muscles, and poorly designed workspaces are often factors in postural stress.

Other factors that can lead to neck pain include:

- Poor posture
- Obesity
- Weak abdominal muscles
- Stress and emotional tension
- Osteoarthritis - progressive deterioration of cartilage
- Spinal stenosis – narrowing of the nerve passageways
- Degenerative disc disease - reduction in the elasticity and height of intervertebral discs
- Whiplash

Studies Show
Single Adjustment Helps Neck Pain

A study published in the September 2006 issue of the Journal of Manipulative and Physiological Therapeutics showed that even just one chiropractic adjustment could help neck pain. In fact, within five minutes of an adjustment, patients have less pain and a better range of motion.[10]

Chiropractic care has been proven to be extremely beneficial to patients suffering from neck pain and it is widely recognized as one of the safest non-invasive therapies available for neck pain complaints. A chiropractor understands that the neck is just one part of the spine and that other symptoms such as shoulder or arm pain are part of the same underlying issue.

Studies Show
Chiropractic Care Beneficial for Chronic Neck Pain

A study published in the February 2006 issue of the Journal of Manipulative and Physiological Therapeutics (JMPT) shows that patients with chronic neck pain benefit from chiropractic. Patients were divided into two groups – one with chiropractic care and one without. Those that received chiropractic care showed significantly less pain intensity. Additionally, Head repositioning accuracy (HRA), a test that measures the ability to reposition the head in a neutral posture after active movements, also showed significant improvement. The conclusion: "The results of this study suggest that chiropractic care can be effective in influencing the complex process of proprioceptive sensibility and pain of cervical origin." In layman's terms, chiropractic can help people with chronic neck pain. [11]

Is It My Heart?

Stat Fact

In a study of 250 patients hospitalized for chest pain, 23% of the non-cardiac patients were felt to have a Costo-sternal cause.[12]

Before beginning this section, I want to be sure that you understand that chest pain can be serious. In fact, it is better to assume that you are having a heart attack and go directly to the emergency room.

However, if after visiting the ER or a cardiologist you find that you are not having cardiovascular issues, you may want to consider chiropractic care. Why? Because nearly one-fourth of chest pain comes from something called costo-sternal chest pain. This pain is due to a subluxation of the costo-chondral cartilage - the joint between the rib and the breastbone.

A subluxated rib head - where the rib joins the spine - can also cause chest pain. Three small joints join the rib to the spine and are easily sprained, even by something as simple as an explosive sneeze. You can tell if you have a subluxated rib head if you have pain when you inhale deeply. This pain often feels like a knife between the shoulder blades.

There is also Thoracic Outlet Syndrome (TOS). With TOS, a large group of nerves called the brachial plexus is affected, causing pain, tingling, or a dull ache in an arm, as well as over the chest and shoulder area. It is caused from a subluxation of the first rib.

As you can see, many people with chest pain actually have a subluxation problem rather than a heart problem. Chiropractic adjustment has proven to be effective for these conditions.

Are You One of the 90 Percent?

Nearly 90% of Americans suffer from headaches. True, not all suffer from debilitating migraines, but any headache is a sign that something is not right. In fact, having no headaches at all is normal for someone that is truly healthy.

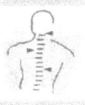 **Words Defined: Migraine**

A severe, disabling headache, usually affecting only one side of the head, and often accompanied by nausea, vomiting, photophobia and visual disturbances.

Headaches can be caused by many different things and are known as triggers. Triggers can include:

- Food
- Noise
- Lights
- Stress
- Muscle tension
- Insomnia
- Excessive exercise
- Blood sugar issues

Ninety-five percent of headaches are just that – headaches. They do not have any underlying disease and are the primary concern. These headaches include tension, migraine or cluster headaches.

The majority of headaches are caused by muscle tension. Americans spend large amounts of time sitting in one position. This causes joint irritation and muscle tension in the neck, upper back, and scalp, causing your neck to ache.

Chiropractors understand how tension in the spine relates to other parts of the body, including those that cause headaches. We can take the necessary steps to relieve headaches for most patients without using drugs.

Studies Show
Headaches Helped by Chiropractic

In the September 2001 issue of the Journal of Manipulative and Physiological Therapeutics was a report on the effectiveness of chiropractic care for patients with chronic headaches. Results showed that the chiropractic group did better than the massage group, and better than the medication group without all the side effects. The conclusion: chiropractic is one of the most effective avenues of health for headache sufferers.[13]

The Crippling Effects of Arthritis

Arthritis is a painful condition of the joints and cartilage. A cycle of pain and mobility loss is associated with arthritis. It works like this:

1. You have joint pain
2. Joint pain causes you to move less
3. Because you move less, you have less mobility
4. As you lose mobility, your arthritis worsens
5. You have more joint pain
6. And on and on

Chiropractic works against this vicious cycle. Your chiropractor's goal is to improve mobility and eliminate pain through chiropractic adjustments. So the new cycle looks like this:

1. Chiropractic adjustment
2. Increased range of motion with less pain
3. You will move more
4. Movement slows or halts the advancement of arthritis
5. Chiropractic adjustment
6. Increased mobility
7. And on and on

Stat Fact

An estimated 46 million adults in the United States reported being told by a doctor that they have some form of arthritis, rheumatoid arthritis, gout, lupus or fibromyalgia. By 2030, an estimated 67 million of Americans aged 18 years or older will have doctor-diagnosed arthritis. [14]

Arthritis puts your body into a negative feedback loop. Chiropractic helps get your body into a positive feedback loop.

Remember, the model for chiropractic is the wellness model and the understanding that the body can heal itself. By correcting subluxations, the chiropractor can increase the range of motion and allow the healing process to begin.

A big benefit of using chiropractic is that you will not have to rely on prescription pain medicines or over-the-counter pain medications with their harmful side effects. Chiropractic is non-invasive and can help arthritis, not as a series of symptoms to be masked, but in a way that will create freedom of movement.

Chiropractic emphasizes the body's ability to heal itself, working through the nervous system, the primary coordinator of all body functions. Studies have shown that chiropractors are helpful in dealing with low back pain, sciatica, neck pain and other chronic pain issues. If you or someone you love has chronic pain, seeing a chiropractor may well be the first step towards health.

SOURCES:

1. *Chronic Pain Management,* Michael E. Schatman, Alexandra Campbell, John D. Loeser. 2007.

2. American Pain Foundation, http://www.painfoundation.org/page.asp?file=Newsroom/PainFacts.htm.

3. K. Beyerman, M. Palmerino, L. Zohn, G. Kane, K. Foster. *Journal of Manipulative and Physiological Therapeutics.* " Efficacy of Treating Low Back Pain and Dysfunction Secondary to Osteoarthritis: Chiropractic Care Compared With Moist Heat Alone." January 2005.

4. K.Hoiriis, B.Pfleger, F.McDuffie, G.Cotsonis, O.Elsangak, R.Hinson, G.Verzosa. *Journal of Manipulative and Physiological Therapeutics.* "A Randomized Clinical Trial Comparing Chiropractic Adjustments to Muscle Relaxants for Subacute Low Back Pain." July 2004.

5. Literature review, Journal of Manipulative and Physiological Therapeutics. March/April 2007.

6. "Chiropractic: An Introduction." *National Center for Complementary & Alternative Medicine.* N.p., n.d. Web.

7. Mitchell Haas, Rajiv Sharma, Miron Stano. *Journal of Manipulative and Physiological Therapeutics* "Cost-Effectiveness of Medical and Chiropractic Care for Acute and Chronic Low Back Pain. October 2005.

8. Blue Cross/Blue Shield (BCBS) of Kansas. "Lumbago Treatment." August 1999.

9. Sanjeeb Shrestha, Pankaj Jay Pasricha. *Digestive Diseases,* "Update on Noncardiac Chest Pain." 2000.

10. R. Martínez-Segura, C. Fernández-de-las-Peñas, M. Ruiz-Sáez, C. López-Jiménez, C. Rodríguez-Blanco. *Journal of Manipulative and Physiological Therapeutics.* "Immediate Effects on Neck Pain and Active Range of Motion After a Single Cervical High-Velocity Low-Amplitude Manipulation in Subjects Presenting with Mechanical Neck Pain: A Randomized Controlled Trial." September 2006.

11. P. Palmgren, P. Sandström, F. Lundqvist, H. Heikkilä. *Journal of Manipulative and Physiological Therapeutics.* "Improvement After Chiropractic Care in Cervicocephalic Kinesthetic Sensibility and Subjective Pain Intensity in Patients with Nontraumatic Chronic Neck Pain." February 2006.

12. National Center for Chronic Disease Prevention and Health Promotion, http://www.cdc.gov/ARTHRITIS/data_statistics/arthritis_related_statistics.htm#1.

13. Gert Bronfort, DC, PhDa, Willem J.J. Assendelft, MD, PhDb, Roni Evans, Dca, Mitchell Haas, DCc, Lex Bouter, PhDd. *Journal of Manipulative and Physiological Therapeutics.* "Efficacy of spinal manipulation for chronic headache: A systematic review." September 2001.

14. NHIS. Arthritis & Rheumatism, 2006

6

CLASS IV LASER AND WARM LASER

Why Dr. Thai Uses Lasers

Dr. Bao Thai uses both Class IV and warm lasers in his practice. Laser therapy is one of the most exciting and amazing discoveries in recent times. It heals and regenerates damaged cells with the use of light energy. Lasers can provide a wonderful array of benefits to help people in pain, help with conditions that take much longer to heal and provide relief to conditions that haven't healed with other modalities.

In the past, chiropractors have used cold lasers or low level lasers (LLLT) for the variety of benefits they provide with their lower power frequencies. Recently, a higher level laser has become popular because of the higher power it provides. The more power, the deeper the laser can reach.

How a Laser Works

Lasers are possible because of the way light interacts with electrons. Electrons exist at specific energy levels or states characteristics of that particular atom or molecule. The energy levels can be imagined as rings or orbits around a nucleus. Electrons in outer rings are at higher energy levels than those in inner rings. Electrons can be bumped up to higher energy levels by the injection of energy – for example, by a flash of light. When an electron drops from an outer to an inner level, "excess" energy is given off as light. The wavelength or color of the emitted light is precisely related to the amount of energy released. Depending on the particular lasing material being used, specific wavelengths of light are absorbed (to energize or excite the electrons) and specific wavelengths are emitted (when the electrons fall back to their initial level).[1]

Class IV Lasers

Lasers stimulate healing at the cellular level. They do this by providing energy to cells through light waves. The wavelength of a class IV laser can penetrate deeply into tissue to change its biochemistry.

When cells lack energy they cannot begin to perform the healing process. In order for cells to heal, the mitochondria of the cell needs to produce a coenzyme called Adenosine triphosphate (ATP), which transports energy.

Interesting Fact

The laser was invented in 1960 and the biostimulative properties of laser light were first discovered in 1967. Therapy lasers have been used in Europe much longer than in the United States. The United States Food and Drug Administration (US FDA) first cleared therapy lasers in 2002, and Class IV lasers in 2003.[2]

A class IV laser and warm laser up to 60 watts uses a wavelength of red light frequency to stimulate the cell, causing it to produce enough ATP so the cell can begin the process of healing the area. When the cells are energized, a chain reaction occurs as they influence other cells increasing *their* energy and the rebuilding of the damaged cells is stimulated. This is healing on a cellular level.

I am one of only a few doctors to offer this treatment in their practice because of the life-changing benefits they provide. Laser therapy is a great option for those who choose it because:

- It is easy to use
- It works quickly
- It is FDA approved
- It is safe
- It is painless
- It feels comfortable to the patient
- It provides quick results
- It has no side effects
- It provides faster healing of conditions
- It speeds recovery time after surgery
- It decreases inflammation

Interesting Fact

The basic science behind deep tissue laser therapy is compelling. Cells absorb the light and undergo significant positive changes. Studies have shown that impaired cells have a stronger response than healthy cells, so the light seems to produce the most benefit where it is most needed.

Lasers work by impacting cellular function. Damaged cells will absorb and become energized by photonic energy; this has been well documented with over 2,000 clinical studies stretching back 30 years. Stimulated cells increase Adenosine triphosphate (ATP) production, and dramatically reduce inflammation, pain and swelling. This modality may be considered a "healing" process, as it quickly corrects compromised cellular function, allowing the body to heal itself.[3]

Benefits of Laser Therapy

When using a class IV laser or warm laser , doctors are often able to treat patients at a faster pace without surgery or drugs. This type of laser uses dual wavelength and dual frequencies to penetrate as deep as four inches into the musculoskeletal tissues.

The laser increases circulation and blood flow, and increases the supply of water, oxygen and nutrients to the damaged area, which in turn stimulates those cells to begin the healing process.

This will reduce:

- Inflammation
- Swelling
- Muscle spasms
- Stiffness
- Pain

Class IV lasers:

- Promote healing
- Improve nerve function
- Reduce scar tissue
- Increase blood flow
- Relieve pain
- Speed up recovery
- Reduce fibrous tissue formation
- Increase metabolic activity
- Improve vascular activity

Research & Science: A Case Study

Lasers have unique wavelengths, which are absorbed by tissues differently. All exhibit the unique qualities of monochronicity and coherence, or the ability of light waves to travel in parallel and phase to give laser energy direction and penetration. In multiple studies, therapeutic lasers have been shown to promote musculoskeletal tissue healing.

Laser therapy promotes healing from a variety of mechanisms known as laser photobiomodulation by photon absorption at a cellular level by photoreceptors or chromophores. The anti-inflammatory properties of therapeutic laser have been shown to follow multiple pathways.[4]

What Conditions Can It Treat?

Different power settings are used to treat different ailments. These settings have different frequencies and wavelengths and because of the versatility of this type of laser, a chiropractor can target specific tissue types which incorporate other factors such as bone, cartilage, connective tissue, muscles, blood vessels and more.[4]

These different power settings enables us to treat musculoskeletal structures such as:

- Neck
- Shoulders

- Back
- Hips
- Wrists
- Elbows
- Knees
- Feet and ankles

The laser can alleviate pain from or heal conditions causing:

- Lower back problems
- Disk related problems (herniated discs, degenerative disc disease)
- Sciatica
- Stenosis
- Strains
- Sprains
- Chronic soreness
- Neuralgias
- Headaches
- TMJ
- Scar tissue
- Bone spurs
- Joint pains
- Arthritic (fingers, toes, ankles)
- Tendonitis
- Bursitis
- Carpal tunnel
- Heavy joints (knees, hips)
- Plantar fasciitis
- Sport injuries

Class IV lasers can even benefit skin conditions including:

- Psoriasis
- Eczema
- Skin lesions
- Herpes
- Shingles
- Toe fungus/athletes foot

Interesting Fact

Most bacteria are anaerobes that proliferate and metabolize much better in the absence of oxygen. Fortunately, this is in direct contradiction with the way our cells flourish and so stimulating the oxygen intake and conversion process will simultaneously help our healthy cells and inhibit bacteria.[5]

How Many Treatments Do I Need?

The success rate of the Class IV laser and warm laser therapy is very high. This type of therapy can be used to assist with post-operative healing, to speed the recovery time and assist with post-surgical pain.

For other conditions that are treated directly with laser therapy, oftentimes patients arrive to their appointment in pain or with limited mobility and after even one treatment have relief, improved mobility and reduced pain.

Interesting Fact

Thermal heat dilates, or expands, blood vessels and increases blood circulation. This, in turn, helps facilitate the healing process. Infrared heat therapy aids in promoting greater tissue flexibility, reduces inflammation and decreases joint pain. This type of therapy is beneficial for many ailments including, arthritis, back pain, Fibromyalgia and tendinitis. Light therapy has also been shown to generate vitamin D in the body.[6]

Most conditions require repeated applications and this depends upon the condition being treated, the severity of the condition and how long the patient has suffered from it. For many people the results are noticeable and remarkable.

What Is the Procedure for Laser Treatments?

When you are having a laser treatment, your chiropractor or practitioner will set the laser for the appropriate wattage for your specific condition. The laser will either be placed on the skin or just above the skin and moved over the area that requires treatment. Laser therapy is applied with constant and/or pulse settings.

No preparation is necessary when having a treatment.

The patient may feel some heat or warmth during the laser treatment and it will not be uncomfortable. In fact, often the patent does not feel anything at all.

Both patient and practitioner (and anyone within the range of the laser) will wear protective goggles for safety purposes.

The treatment time can vary depending upon the size of the area being treated. Treatment ranges between five minutes to 20 minutes depending upon the size of the area(s) being treated.

In Conclusion

Class IV lasers and warm laser are an amazing new tool for health benefits in every area of the medical world. Chiropractors are increasing their services to patients by combining the use of these lasers with their regular treatment process.

With the speed and benefit of healing new or chronic injuries with laser treatment, the possibilities are endless. This is one of the most exciting innovations to hit the medical field and it is worth investigating if you suffer from any ailment previously mentioned. Just ask your chiropractor how class IV lasers can benefit you.

Studies Show
Class IV Laser and warm laser Therapy Interventional and Case Reports Confirm Positive Therapeutic Outcomes in Multiple Clinical Indications

Tissue that is damaged and poorly oxygenated as a result of swelling, trauma or inflammation has been shown to respond significantly to laser therapy irradiation. At the cellular level, deep penetrating photons activate a biochemical cascade of events leading to increased DNA/RNA, protein and collagen synthesis, increased CAMP levels, and cellular proliferation. The result of these reactions is rapid cellular regeneration, normalization and healing.

Laser light energy is highly absorbed by skin and subcutaneous tissue, therefore, penetration is key to therapeutic result. Longer wavelengths and higher power output result in deeper penetration and higher dosage to the tissue. Larger laser therapeutic dosage levels produce improved clinical outcomes as illustrated in the case and interventional studies cited above. LLLT (Classes I-III) does not provide optimal clinical outcomes in most disease conditions because they cannot deliver the necessary dosage to deep structures without using excessively long treatment times. Class IV lasers and warm laser have been shown to provide both the wavelengths and output power levels necessary to trigger therapeutic cellular metabolic changes.[7]

SOURCES:

1. Bellis, M. "How a Laser Â Works." *About.com Inventors*. N.p., n.d.

2. FAQs & Support." *KLaserUSA FAQs Support Comments*.

3. Santiago, Philip, D.C., and Julie L. Scarano, D.C. "Advances in Sports Chiropractic from the Olympic Athlete to the Weekend Warrior:Class IV Deep Tissue Laser Therapy." *The American Chiropractor* (2010): 22. Web.

4. Frostad, Mike, ATC, Geroge Poulis, MA, ATC, and Glenn Dopeland, DPM. "Major League Relief." *Advance for Directors in Rehabilitation* (2009): n. pag. Web.

5. Knapp, Daniel, DC. *Class IV Laser Therapy Treatment of Multifactorial Lumbar Stenosis With Low-Back and Leg Pain: A Case Report*. Rep. N.p.: K-Laser USA, n.d. Web.

6. Stephens, Bryan J., PhD. "Mechanisms of Action." *KLaserUSA Mechanisms of Action Comments*. N.p., n.d.

7. Romero, Caroline. "Therapeutic Uses for Infrared Heat." *EHow*. Demand Media, 05 Aug. 2010. Web.

8. Pryor, B. PhD., Udel.edu. (Sept. 2009). LiteCure, LLC. Class IV Laser Therapy Interventional and case reports confirm positive therapeutic outcomes in multiple clinical indications. As retrieved from: http://www.udel.edu/PT/PT%20Clinical%20 Services/journalclub/caserounds/11-12/September/ PryorLaserPromotional.pdf

7

REHABILITATION EXERCISES AND STRETCHES

What Is Rehabilitation Exercise?

Rehabilitation exercise helps you to recover from injury or surgery, or reduce symptoms of years of abuse to the spine. In order to understand the need for rehabilitation exercise, let's take a look at the mechanics of the spine.

There are three types of muscles that support the spine:

- **Extensors: They straighten the back, lift and extend, and move the thighs away from the body.**

- **Flexors:** They bend and support the spine from the front. They also control the lower spine and move the thighs toward the body.

- **Obliques or Rotators:** They are used to stabilize the spine when upright. They also rotate the spine and help maintain proper posture and spinal curvature.

All of these muscles weaken with age and many are simply not used enough to perform at their optimal function. Rehabilitative exercises can increase the muscle strength in these three groups to improve your spinal health.

Why Do Rehabilitation Exercises

Exercise rehabilitation is vital for those with chronic disease, injuries or disabilities. It will help improve body function, health and quality of life. There is new evidence showing that even a small injury can take up to a year to heal completely.

When you have been inactive for a long time, it will be difficult to regain your strength. Your joints may become stiff and your muscles weak due to disuse. The longer you remain inactive, the longer it will take to regain your lost strength and return to active living. To get back on your feet again, you need to put your body back to *use* with exercise.

The goal of rehabilitation exercises is to restore range of motion, strength, endurance and to prevent new occurrences, relapses or further progression of a condition. Any kind of injury will cause specific muscles to stop working, or stop working correctly, so it will be essential to retrain muscles.

Your problem may have taken months or even years to occur. Rehabilitation exercises can reverse the degenerative process faster than it occurred, but it may still take several months to be complete. A rehab program usually includes treatment with a chiropractor, as well as home treatment. In general, as you see less of your chiropractor, you do more on your own.

Your therapy will be guided by your chiropractor and designed specifically for you and your issues. This therapy will guide you through exercises to reach your rehab goals taking your health status, age and activity expectations into account.

Be sure to talk with your chiropractor before starting any home exercises. Without his expert guidance, you may end up aggravating or worsening your problem, even if you aren't experiencing pain.

Benefits of Rehabilitation Exercises

We all benefit from the right type of exercise regardless of our injury, age and ability.

There are many benefits to receiving rehabilitative exercise therapy:

- Increased muscle strength and endurance
- Increased range of motion
- Decreased pain
- Decreased swelling and inflammation of joints
- Increased coordination and balance
- Increased mobility
- Improved physical well being and health
- Improved body mechanics and posture
- Decreased stress
- Increased spinal strength and stability
- Increased joint function and flexibility
- Increased function of the ankle, knee and hip as it relates to balance
- Increased response of the core muscles

This is only a small list of the benefits of exercise for health and rehabilitation.

With regular exercise, your level of physical ability and fitness will gradually improve. You will find you have more energy and stamina, and you will receive the additional benefits of improved mental status, appetite, relaxation and sleep at night.

Seniors and Exercise

According to the American College of Sports Medicine, by the year 2030 the number of people in the United States 65 years and over will reach 70 million. Understanding what happens to your body as you age and how exercise can help is important.

Let's first look at muscles. Muscle keeps you strong, it burns calories, and contributes to balance and bone strength. The problem is that muscle mass decreases as you age. As you lose muscle mass, you can also lose your independence and mobility. The good news is that muscle mass can increase at any age in response to exercise.

Studies Show
Seniors Can Rebuild Muscle Mass

Subjects aged 72 to 98 years of age lifted weights with their legs three times a week for 10 weeks. At the end of the study, there was an increase in thigh mass of 2.7%, walking speed increased 12%, and leg strength increased 113%.[1]

Endurance is something else that decreases with age. Studies have shown that the slower a person walks, the more likely they are to suffer from illnesses. But, like with muscle mass, there is something you can do about endurance. Just get out there and walk. In a study of 41,000 men and women from 1990 to 2001, data was analyzed to find the relationship between walking and mortality. Men and women who walked 30 minutes or more per day during the study period had fewer deaths than those who walked less than 30 minutes.[2]

Do you want to guess what happens to flexibility as you age? It decreases. However, once again, exercise can help you improve your flexibility. Several studies of exercise and the aging show that improvements in range of motion of the neck, shoulder, elbow, wrist, hip, knee and ankle occur if doing stretching exercises.

Another thing that decreases when we age is balance. A major result of this decrease is falling. According to the U.S. Centers for Disease Control and Prevention (CDC), one of every three Americans over the age of 65 falls each year, and among individuals 65-84, falls account for 87% of all fractures and are the second leading cause of spinal cord and brain injury.[3] The good news is that physical activity can improve balance and reduce the risk of falling.

It is important to select balance exercises that correspond to your everyday activities. For instance, you may want to work on leg balancing exercises if you are unsteady when you walk.

Another thing that decreases with age is bone density. This can lead to osteoporosis, which in turn leads to a higher risk of bone fracture. According to the National Osteoporosis Foundation, osteoporosis affects 44 million men and women ages 50 and older in the United States, or 55% of the people 50 years of age and older.[4]

Studies are now showing that weight lifting and even simple walking can increase bone density in the hip and spine. This happens because these activities cause stress on the bone, which stimulates them to grow.

Another system that has problems as we age is the joints. Many older adults have osteoarthritis. Exercise can improve function for people with arthritis.

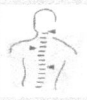 **Words Defined: Osteoarthritis**

Arthritis that affects the bone by wearing down the cushion that pads the space between bones.

Another benefit of exercise is increased cognitive function. Neurons, those cells that help you think, move and memorize, increase after a few short weeks of exercise. Studies have shown that the fittest seniors have the most brain tissue and this helped them with activities such as coordination, scheduling, planning and memory.

Finally, exercise can help you increase your mood. Many seniors, upwards of 20% of those over 55, are depressed. Exercise can alleviate the symptoms of depression.

What does all this mean to you? The benefits of exercise abound, so get out there and get moving!

Three Types of Rehabilitative Exercise

There are three types of rehabilitative exercise: stretching, strength training and low-impact aerobics.

Stretching helps you to push your range of motion in a controlled manner. As you increase your mobilization, you will also reduce associated pain in your spine. The goal of stretching is to achieve flexibility and elasticity in the disk, muscles, ligaments and tendons.

Strength training is exercising with the goal of increasing your physical strength. Strength training increases endurance and bone density. It strengthens your joints, lowers cholesterol and improves your sleep. Future episodes of back pain are less likely to occur if back strengthening is used along with stretching.

Finally, conditioning through low-impact aerobic exercise is very important for both rehabilitation and maintenance of the lower back. Examples of low impact aerobic exercise that many people with back pain can tolerate include pool therapy, walking and stationary biking.

Choosing the most appropriate form of exercise depends upon the nature of the injury and an individual's exercise preferences. Your chiropractor can help you choose an exercise program that will work best for you.

Low-Tech Exercises

Low-tech exercises include stretches, range of motion and strength training without using any special equipment. Here are a few that are good for the neck and back.

Exercises to Do While Lying on Your Back

Pelvic Tilt: This stretches the back muscles and strengthens the stomach muscles. Lie on your back with your knees bent and your feet flat on the floor. Rest your hands on your pelvis. Tighten your abdomen and buttock muscles. Press your lower back onto the floor (a small and subtle movement). Hold 5 seconds, release.

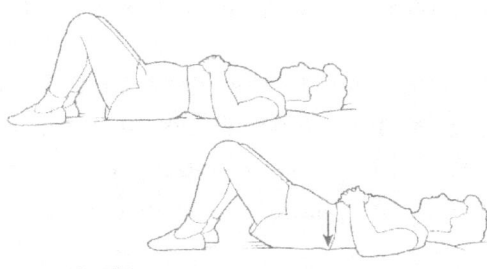

Lower Back Rotation: This stretches and strengthens the back rotation muscles. Once again, live on your back with your knees bent and your feet flat on the floor. Drop both knees to one side while rotating your head to the opposite side. Hold 5 seconds. Alternate sides.

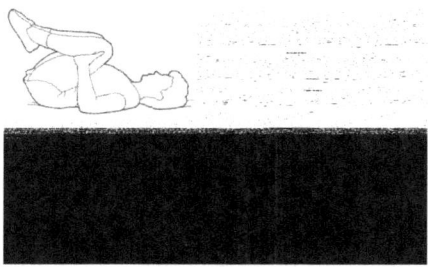

Double Leg Pull: This stretches the lower back and buttock muscles. Gently pull both knees to your chest. Hold 5 seconds, then return to the start position.

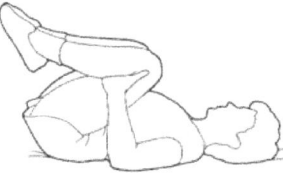

Hip Lift: Strengthens the buttock muscles. Without arching your back, slowly raise your hips upward. Make it a straight line from knees to shoulders. Hold for 5 seconds.

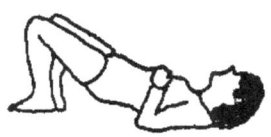

Single Leg Pull: Stretches the hip, lower back and buttock muscles. Slowly pull a bent knee to your chest while keeping the other knee and the lower back pressed against the floor. Hold for 5 seconds. Alternate legs.

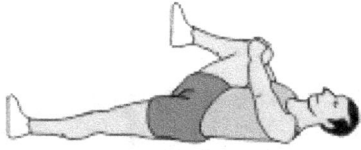

Straight Leg Raise: Stretches the hips and hamstring muscles, and strengthens the quadriceps muscles. Keeping your lower back pressed against the floor, raise the straight leg until it's level with the bent knee. Hold for 5 seconds. Alternate legs.

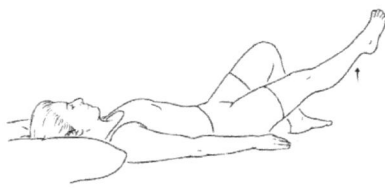

Partial Curl Ups: Strengthens abdominal muscles. Lying on your back with your knees bent and feet flat on the floor, cross your arms loosely and tuck your chin in. Tighten your abdomen and curl halfway up directly in front of you. Hold for 5 seconds.

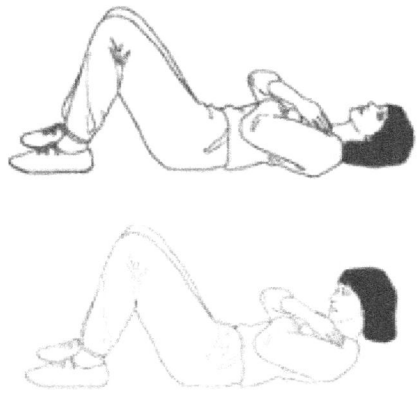

Exercises To Do On Your Hands and Knees

Back Press: This exercise strengthens abdominal muscles and buttocks and stretches your back. Start on your hands and knees. Keep your stomach firm and do not arch your back or let it sag. This is called a neutral position. Keep your ears aligned with your shoulders. Press your back upward by tightening your abdominal and buttock muscles at the same time. Allow your head to drop slightly keeping your hands and knees still. Hold for 5 seconds.

Back Release: This stretches your back muscles. Do this in conjunction with the back press. Allow your stomach and the muscles of your buttocks to relax and let your back sag. Hold for 5 seconds.

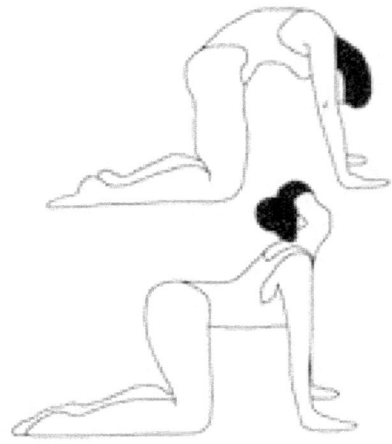

Arm Reach: Strengthens your shoulders and upper back. While on your hands and knees, stretch one arm straight out in front of you. Don't raise your head and don't let your back sag. Hold for 5 seconds. Alternate arms.

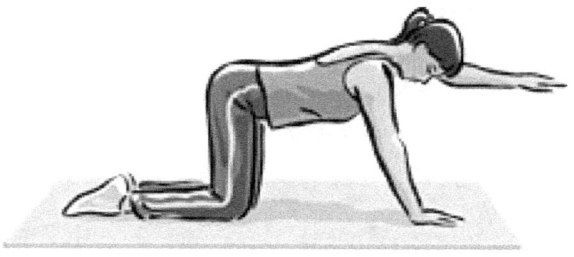

Leg Reach: Strengthens the muscles of your buttocks. Extend one leg straight out behind you and hold it parallel to the floor for 5 seconds without letting your head, back or stomach sag. Alternate legs.

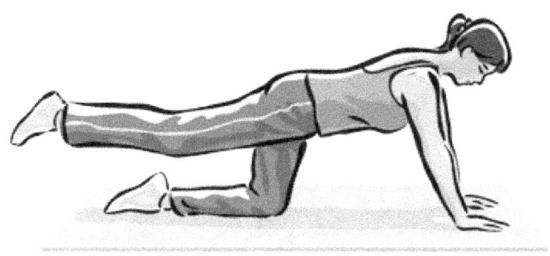

Exercises To Do Standing Up

Wall Slide: Strengthens the back, hip and leg muscles. With your back against the wall, legs slightly apart, sink straight down slowly as if sitting in a chair. Hold for 5 seconds.

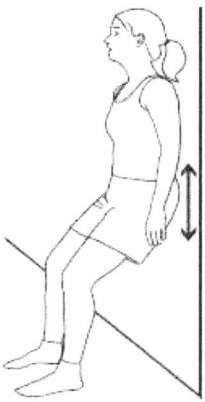

Calf Stretch: Stretches the calf muscles. Feet slightly apart, bend your front leg, keeping the heel of your back foot firmly on the floor. Lean forward. You can grasp a chair, or table if needed. Hold 30 seconds. Alternate legs.

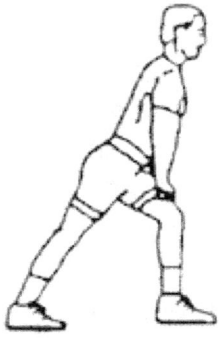

Hamstring Stretch: Stretches the hamstrings and lower back. Put one foot up on a chair. Keep the elevated leg and back straight, bend forward slowly as if trying to meet your knee with your head. Hold for 5 seconds. Alternate legs.

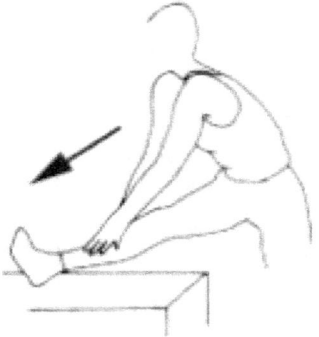

Side Stretch: Stretches the muscles in your back and side. Stretch your arm overhead and slowly bend to the opposite side. Don't twist. Hold 5 seconds, return to start. Alternate sides.

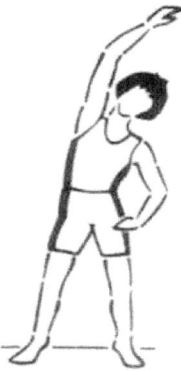

Shoulder Shrug: Stretches and strengthens the shoulder and upper back muscles. Raise both of your shoulders as high as you can, as if you were trying to touch your ears. Hold for 5 seconds.

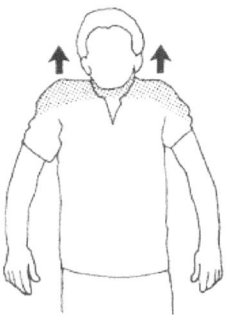

Standing Back Stretch: Stretches and strengthens lower back. Stand with feet shoulder length apart and place your hands in the small of your back. Bend back slowly, as far as tolerated, while keeping your knees straight. Hold for 5 seconds.

Rehabilitative Exercise Equipment

In addition to doing simple exercises, your chiropractor may have you perform exercises using specialized rehabilitation equipment.

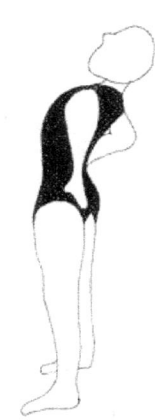

Exercise balls: These balls help improve balance, coordination, flexibility, strength and sense of relative position. An exercise ball is used, rather than the floor or a wall, in order to engage more muscles. Your body must respond to the unsteadiness of the ball to remain balanced. Typically, your core muscles (those in the abdomen and back) are the focus of exercise ball exercises.

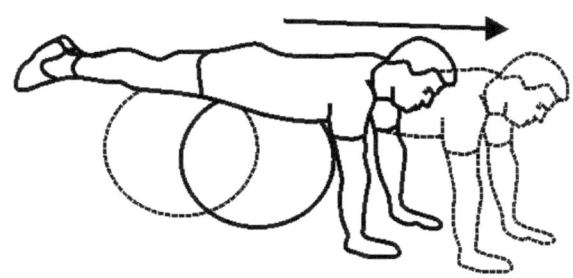

Resistance exercisers: Resistance bands are used in strength training exercise. They look like giant rubber bands and help you to strengthen specific muscle groups. Resistance bands come in a range of resistance levels, from easy-to-stretch to progressively more difficult.

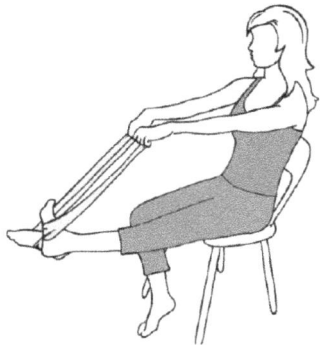

Exercise bikes: A stationary bike is a low-impact aerobic option that is easy on your joints. There are two main types of exercise bikes:

- Upright bike: This bike sits like a regular bike with your legs extended below your torso.
- Recumbent bike: This bike is more like a chair, with support on your back and your legs extended in front of you.

What's nice about using an exercise bike versus a regular bike is that you can manually control your workout incline, resistance and speed.

Treadmills or stairmaster; These are the motorized version of walking or running in place. You keep up with a belt that's moving under your feet. Treadmill workouts burn about the same number of calories as walking or running outdoors.

Balance boards: These are also called wobble boards. The main goal of a balance board is to improve your sense and awareness of the position of your body parts. This is called proprioception, which helps to reduce the risk of injury. You can also use the board to improve stability, enhance your strength, train for specific board sports and for physical rehabilitation.

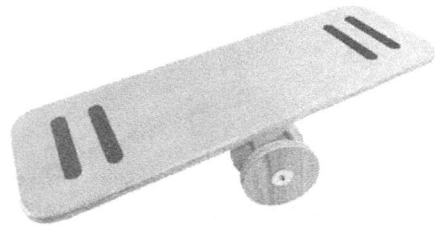

Rebounders: You may know this piece of equipment as a mini-trampoline or a Bosu balance ball These are therapy devices that will help you with balance and rebounding. **They can improve your coordination and promote increased muscle tone.** Rebounders provide an all-over body workout.

SOURCES:

1. "Influence of Resistance Exercise on Lean Body Mass in Aging Adults: A Meta-Analysis," *Medicine & Science in Sports & Exercise.* 2010.

2. van der Bij AK, Laurent MGH, Wensing M. "Effectiveness of physical activity interventions for older adults: a review." American Journal of Preventative Medicine. 2002.

3. Centers for Disease Control and Prevention. "Falls Among Older Adults." http://www.cdc.gov/ HomeandRecreationalSafety/Falls/adultfalls.html.

4. http://www.nof.org/.

GLOSSARY

Abdomen: The part of the body between the chest and hips, aka, belly.

Activator® Methods: A small hand-held adjusting instrument which delivers a precisely measured, gentle thrust in a specific direction.

Acute: Comes on quickly, can be severe, but lasts a relatively short time.

Adjustment: A procedure to restore joint mobility, alignment and nerve communication by applying a specific and controlled force to joints by manual or mechanical means.

Afferent: Carrying inward to a central organ or section, as nerves that conduct impulses from the periphery of the body to the brain or spinal cord.

Antalgic Position: Abnormal body position due to the body's attempt to reduce pain.

Anterior: Toward the front of the body.

Articulation: Joining bones to allow motion; a joint.

Atlas: The uppermost, most movable bone of the spine, also referred to as "C1" or Cervical 1, which supports the skull. So named from the Greek God, Atlas, who was said to hold the World on his shoulders.

Atrophy: Partial or complete wasting away of a part of the body.

Autonomic Nervous System (ANS): The part of the nervous system in charge of regulating involuntary vital functions, including the activity of the heart, the digestive system and the glands. It's divided into two subsystems: the sympathetic nervous system and the parasympathetic nervous system.

Axis: The second vertebra in the cervical area of the spinal column, also referred to as C2, is the second level in the cervical spine. So called due to its unusual shape having an odontoid process that serves as an axis for rotation of the C1 or "Atlas".

Bilateral: Having, or relating to, two sides.

Biomechanics: Mechanics applied to biology in order to understand the mechanics of living systems.

Blocks/blocking: Wedge-shaped apparatus used to raise one or both sides of the hip bone into a healthier pattern for better support of the spine and head.

Bursitis: The painful inflammation of the bursa, a pad-like sac found in areas subject to friction. Bursae cushion the movement between the bones, tendons and muscles near the joints.

CAT Scan (Computer Aided Tomography): A series of detailed pictures of areas inside the body, taken from different angles; the 3-D pictures are created by a computer linked to an x-ray machine.

Central Nervous System (CNS): The portion of the vertebrate nervous system consisting of the brain and spinal cord.

Cerebellum: The posterior portion of the brain that plays an important role in motor control. The cerebellum does not initiate movement, but it contributes to , precision, and accurate timing. It receives input from (proprioception) of the spinal cord and from other parts of the , and integrates these inputs to fine tune motor activity. Cerebellar damage does not cause , but instead results in disorders in fine movement, , , and .

Cervical: The upper spinal area, consisting of seven vertebrae. Commonly referred to as the neck.

Chiropractic: The art, science and philosophy which utilizes the inherent recuperative powers of the body and deals with the relationship between the spinal column and nervous system and the role of that relationship in the restoration and maintenance of health.

Chiropractor: Doctor trained in the specific science, art and philosophy of chiropractic.

Chronic: Lasting for a long period of time or marked by frequent recurrence.

Coccyx: A small triangular bone at the base of the spinal column consisting of several fused rudimentary vertebrae.

Compensation Reaction: A problem resulting from the body responding to a problem elsewhere.

Compressive Lesion: A malfunctioning spinal bone or soft tissue that puts direct pressure on a nerve, distorting its function.

Congenital: Present since birth.

CT Scan: See CAT Scan.

Davis Series: Seven specific x-ray views of the upper spine to help with whiplash.

Diagnostic Imaging: Diagnostic imaging includes all tests that produce images or pictures of the inside of the body.

Disc: Also called Intervertebral discs (or intervertebral fibrocartilage); lies between adjacent in the . Each disc forms a cartilaginous to allow slight movement of the vertebrae, and acts as a to hold the vertebrae together. Also, the disc serves as a shock absorber between the vertebrae of the spinal column. Discs consist of a crisscrossing outer layer called the annulus fibrosis and an inner gelatinous portion called the nucleus pulposus.

Disc Herniation: A bulging of the nucleus pulposus into or through the outer layers of the disc called the annulus fibrosis, often causing pain and disc dysfunction both locally and/or in the associated nerves.

Disease: An abnormal condition of the body or mind that causes discomfort or dysfunction.

Dorsal: Pertaining to the back or to the posterior part of an organ; older term for thoracic vertebra, of which there are 12. Thoracic vertebra or "dorsals" are unique in that they are the only normal vertebrae that have ribs attached.

Efferent: Refers to nerves that carry messages from the brain and spinal cord towards the muscles and glands in the body, i.e. motor nerves.

Electromyogram (EMG): A graphical record of electric currents associated with muscle contractions.

Electro-Muscle Stimulation (EMS): A therapeutic type of electrical current applied directly to the body and used for the relief of pain, swelling and inflammation, muscle spasm and to heal injured tissue.

Extension: To stretch or spread something out to greater or fullest length; in anatomical terms, moving in a backward or posterior direction when referring to the spine and moving the limb away from the body when referring to the extremities.

Facet: A smooth flat surface at the posterior of each vertebra that links them with vertebra above and below and permits movement of the spine.

Facilitative Lesion: A twisting, stretching, chafing or irritation of nerve tissue from malfunctioning spinal structures.

Fixation: Spinal area with restricted movement.

Flaccid: Lacking firmness, resilience or muscle tone; drooping.

Flexion: The act of bending a joint or limb in the body towards the body, regarding the spine – bending forward.

Foramen: An opening or orifice, as in a bone.

Health: A state of optimal physical, mental, and social well-being and not merely the absence of disease and infirmity.

Homeostasis: A body's ability to regulate in order to achieve a relatively stable state of equilibrium.

Hypermobility: A condition in which the joints easily move beyond the normal range expected for a particular joint.

Hypertonicity: The abnormal state of high muscle tone; too much tension or tightness in a muscle, often resulting in decreased circulation and in severe cases can cause cell death due to lack of oxygen.

Hypomobility: Condition in which ligaments are tight and movement is restricted.

Hypoxia: "Hypo" meaning "less than" or "under" and "oxia" referring to oxygen (O_2). Hypoxia is a state of decreased or limited oxygen in tissues. Muscular hypoxia can occur secondary to muscle spasm or increased tension in the muscles.

Inflammation: A localized protective reaction of tissue to irritation, injury, or infection, characterized by pain, redness, swelling and sometimes loss of function.

Interference: Damage or deficit to the natural nerve flow.

Intervertebral Disc: The soft tissue found between the bones of the spinal column, i.e. the vertebrae. They help cushion the spine from everyday stress.

Intervertebral Foramina: The two narrow spaces between adjacent vertebrae (one on each side), through which nerve roots pass.

Kyphosis: A normal curvature of the spine when in the thoracic region.

Lateral: To the side of the midline of the body.

Listing: A way to describe the way vertebral segments are in relation to adjacent vertebral segments.

Lordosis: A normal inward (forward) curvature of the vertebral column when in the cervical and lumbar regions.

Lumbar: The five vertebrae that are situated in the lower back region, below the thoracic vertebrae and above the sacral vertebrae in the spinal column.

Massage: A manual therapeutic modality of the body that increases circulation, reduces muscle spasm and promotes relaxation and well-being.

Magnetic Resonance Imaging (MRI): An imaging technique that uses magnetic forces to obtain detailed images of the body.

Mechanoreceptor - Cells specialized to detect and transmit mechanical stimuli and relay that information centrally in the nervous system. Mechanoreceptors are involved with postural balance and proprioception.

Neural Canal: A canal formed by neural arches of vertebrae. Houses the spinal cord.

Neurological: Having to do with the brain, spinal cord and nerves, i.e. the nervous system.

Nucleus Pulposus: The jelly-like substance in the middle of the spinal disc.

Objective Complaints: Areas of concern found through chiropractic examination.

Orthopedics: The science of prevention, diagnosis and treatment of diseases and abnormalities of musculoskeletal systems.

Palpation: Examining the spine with your fingers; the art of feeling with the hands.

Pathophysiology: The physiological processes associated with disease or injury.

Peripheral Nerve System (PNS): The section of the nervous system lying outside the brain and spinal cord. Cells of the peripheral nervous system carry information to and from the central nervous system.

Physiology: The study of the physical and chemical processes involved in the functioning of the human body.

Posterior: Toward the back of the body.

Postural Balance: A posture in which an ideal body mass distribution is achieved. Postural balance provides the body carriage stability and conditions for normal functions in stationary position or in movement, such as sitting, standing or walking.

Preventive Care: Comprehensive care emphasizing priorities for prevention, early detection and early treatment of conditions.

Prognosis: A prediction of the future course of a condition or illness based on scientific study.

Prone: Lying face downward.

Proprioception: "Individual perception" or the unconscious sense of the body to determine how it is positioned in space and the strength of effort being employed in movement. Proprioception provides sense of stationary positions and movements of one's body parts, and is important in maintaining kinesthesia and postural balance. It is provided by **proprioceptors** in and in . The cerebellum is largely responsible for coordinating the unconscious aspects of proprioception.

Radiograph: A film with an image of body tissues that was produced when the body was placed adjacent to the film while radiating with x-rays.

Range of Motion: A measurement of the extent to which a joint can go through all of its normal movements.

Reflex: An involuntary and almost instant movement in response to stimulus.

Rib: The long curved bones that start at the spinal column and form the rib cage, which encloses the lungs and heart. Humans have 24 ribs (12 on each side) and there is a nerve (intercostal nerve) that travels in a groove on the bottom side of the rib. Any misalignment of the rib that causes deformation of the intercostal nerve can cause severe pain and difficulty taking a deep breath. Can mimic a heart attack.

Sacrum: A large triangular bone located between the two hipbones and formed from fused vertebrae.

Scar Tissue – soft tissue fibrosis; an area of fibrosis often found in muscles that have been damaged or overused that can result in spot welds between muscles and contractures within the muscles.

Sciatica: An inflammation of the sciatic nerve, usually marked by pain and tenderness along the course of the nerve through the gluteal region, thigh and leg.

Scoliosis: Sideways (lateral) curving of the spine.

Slipped Disc: Incorrect name for disc herniation.

Spasm: A painful and involuntary muscular contraction.

Spinous Process: A bony projection of a vertebra that serves as an attachment for muscles and ligaments.

Spurring: Any sharply pointed projection, as from a bone.

Subjective Complaints: Problems identified by the patient and reported to the doctor, such as lower back pain, aching joints, etc.

Subluxation: An interference of the nervous system due to a misalignment and or abnormal motion of spinal vertebra which causes improper communication with associated organs, muscles and tissues of the body.

Superior: Upper or higher in position.

Supine: Lying on the back.

Technique: A practical method or procedure applied to correct spinal problems.

Therapy: Methods used to assist in the relief of pain, rehabilitation and restoration of normal body functions.

Thoracic: The region of the spine between the neck and the lumbar vertebrae. The ribs connect with the 12 thoracic vertebrae.

Transverse Process: The lateral bony wings projecting from the side of the vertebrae for muscle attachment.

Trigger Point: A taut, palpable spot in muscle that is painful to touch and refers pain to another body area.

Ultrasound: High frequency sounds beyond a human's hearing whose vibrations can be used for heating internal structures of the body to speed the healing of a joint, muscle or tendon.

Vertebra: One of the bony segments of the spinal column.

Vertebral Subluxation: See Subluxation.

Wellness Care: Health care that is not prompted by sickness or injury but by an attempt to achieve or promote an optimum state of physical, mental and social well-being.

Whiplash: Injury resulting from a sudden sharp whipping movement of the neck and head, such as with a person in a vehicle that is struck from the rear by another vehicle.

X-rays: Electromagnetic radiation that can penetrate many objects and reveal their internal structure by recording the shadow cast on photographic plates; common term for the radiographs that are produced using X-rays. Most X-ray images are recorded in digital images currently.

Zen Stretch™: Dr. Kim's explanation of the proper way to dynamically stretch injured or shortened muscle tissues without engaging the muscle's natural defense mechanisms by doing a series of slow movements with breathing and pauses to allow the muscle to unwind.